# DMSO Guide Made Easy for Beginners

## Understanding the Science of DMSO

By

Conall Dorian

Copyright@2023

# Table of Contents


CHAPTER 1 ........................................5

Introduction .....................................5

1.1 What is DMSO ........................5

1.2 History and Discovery ..............6

1.3 Common Uses and Applications
........................................................8

CHAPTER 2 ......................................12

Understanding the Science of DMSO
........................................................12

2.1 Chemical Structure and
Properties ......................................12

2.2 How DMSO Works ................18

2.3 Safety Considerations .............23

CHAPTER 3 ......................................30

Getting Started with DMSO ............30

3.1 Handling and Storage .............30

3.2 Dilution and Concentration ....36

CHAPTER 4 ......................................42

DMSO as a Solvent ......................42

4.1 Using DMSO as a Solvent .....42

4.2 Mixing DMSO with Other
Substances ................................47

4.3 Compatibility with Different
Compounds...............................53

CHAPTER 5 ................................60

DMSO's Therapeutic Potential........60

5.1 Medical and Pharmaceutical
Applications ..............................61

5.2 Topical and Transdermal Uses
...................................................64

5.3 Safety and Precautions in
Therapeutic Applications .............66

CHAPTER 6 ................................74

DMSO in Research and Industry.....74

6.1 Scientific Research and Lab
Applications ..............................74

6.2 Industrial and Manufacturing
Uses .........................................78

6.3 Environmental Considerations
.......................................................81

# CHAPTER 1

# Introduction

## 1.1 What is DMSO

Dimethyl sulfoxide, commonly known as DMSO, is an organic solvent with a remarkable range of properties and applications. It is a colorless, odorless, and highly polar liquid that was first synthesized in 1866 by a Russian scientist named Alexander Zaytsev. Its unique characteristics and versatility have made it a subject of significant interest and investigation in various fields, ranging from chemistry and biology to medicine and industry.

At its core, DMSO is a powerful solvent. It possesses the ability to dissolve a wide array of organic and inorganic compounds, which is attributed to its highly polar nature and its capacity to mix both with polar and nonpolar substances. This property makes it an invaluable tool in research, as it can help scientists dissolve and manipulate substances that may be otherwise insoluble in water or other common solvents.

## 1.2 History and Discovery

The history of DMSO is a fascinating journey that starts with its accidental discovery in the mid-19th century. While DMSO's chemical structure was first synthesized by Alexander Zaytsev in 1866, its potential uses remained largely unexplored until the mid-20th century. In 1961, Stanley

W. Jacob, a researcher at the
University of Oregon Medical School,
began studying the compound for its
potential medical applications.

Jacob's work led to the realization that
DMSO had not only remarkable
solvent properties but also
demonstrated unique properties as a
transdermal carrier, enabling the
delivery of substances through the
skin. This breakthrough opened up an
entirely new realm of possibilities in
medicine, which included the
treatment of various inflammatory
and painful conditions. However, it's
important to note that DMSO's
journey was not without controversy,
and its approval and use in medicine
remain the subject of debate and
regulation in various countries.

# 1.3 Common Uses and Applications

DMSO's versatility has led to its widespread use across various fields. Here are some common uses and applications of DMSO:

**Laboratory and Research:**

- DMSO serves as a versatile solvent in the laboratory, facilitating the dissolution of a wide range of compounds for chemical analyses, spectroscopy, and crystallization.

- It is used in cryopreservation to store biological samples at extremely low temperatures without damaging the cell structures.

**Medical and Pharmaceutical:**

- DMSO has been investigated for its potential in treating various medical conditions, including arthritis, interstitial cystitis, and chronic pain.

- In certain cases, it has been used as a transdermal carrier to deliver medications through the skin.

- Its anti-inflammatory properties have led to exploration in the field of sports medicine and rehabilitation.

**Industrial and Manufacturing:**

- DMSO is employed as a solvent in the production of various chemicals and polymers.

- It is used in the manufacturing of electronics and other high-tech products.

- In the production of adhesives and coatings, DMSO serves as a valuable component.

**Veterinary:**

- DMSO has found applications in veterinary medicine, particularly in the treatment of injuries and inflammations in animals.

**Alternative and Complementary Therapies:**

- DMSO has been embraced by proponents of alternative and complementary medicine for various therapeutic purposes, although its use in this context is often controversial.

DMSO, with its intriguing history and wide-ranging applications, is a compound that continues to captivate the scientific and medical communities. Its unique properties make it a valuable tool for research and innovation across a multitude of domains, despite the ongoing discussions surrounding its regulation and safety. As we delve deeper into this guide, we will explore the science behind DMSO, its safe usage, and the various applications in greater detail.

# CHAPTER 2

# Understanding the Science of DMSO

## 2.1 Chemical Structure and Properties

Dimethyl sulfoxide (DMSO) is a fascinating compound with a unique chemical structure and a diverse range of properties that make it valuable in various fields. Understanding the science of DMSO begins with examining its chemical structure and inherent properties.

**Chemical Structure:**

DMSO is an organosulfur compound with the chemical formula $(CH_3)_2SO$. Its molecular structure features a sulfur atom (S) bonded to two methyl groups (CH3) and one oxygen atom (O) in a tetrahedral arrangement. The key features of its chemical structure include:

- **Sulfur-Oxygen Double Bond:** The sulfur atom is double-bonded to the oxygen atom, creating a sulfoxide group. This double bond is critical to DMSO's reactivity and unique properties.

- **Methyl Groups:** Two methyl (CH3) groups are attached to the sulfur atom. These groups contribute to the compound's overall structure and affect its solubility and reactivity.

**Physical Properties:**

DMSO exhibits several noteworthy physical properties that influence its practical applications:

- **Physical State:** DMSO is a colorless liquid at room temperature and is often described as odorless or having a faint garlic-like odor. Its liquid state and lack of color make it an ideal solvent in various applications.

- **Solvent Properties:** DMSO's most famous attribute is its remarkable solvency. It is an excellent solvent for a wide range of organic and inorganic substances. It can dissolve polar and nonpolar compounds, which is due to its high polarity, making it a versatile tool in research and industry.

- **High Boiling Point:** DMSO has a relatively high boiling point of around 189°C (372°F). This high boiling point makes it suitable for applications that require elevated temperatures for dissolving or processing compounds.

- **Hygroscopic Nature:** DMSO is hygroscopic, meaning it readily absorbs moisture from the surrounding environment. This property can affect the concentration of DMSO solutions over time, necessitating careful storage and handling.

- **Viscosity:** DMSO has a higher viscosity compared to many other solvents. This viscosity can influence its flow and mixing properties in various applications.

## Chemical Properties:

DMSO's chemical properties contribute to its reactivity and versatility:

- **Reactivity:** DMSO is a highly reactive compound. It can act as a nucleophile, participating in various chemical reactions. Its sulfur atom can form bonds with electrophilic molecules, making it valuable in both synthesis and dissolution processes.

- **Stability:** DMSO is generally stable under standard conditions, but it may undergo reactions or degradation in specific situations. Understanding its stability is essential when using DMSO in various applications to ensure safety and effectiveness.

- **Odor:** While pure DMSO is described as odorless, it can develop a garlic-like odor when exposed to air. This odor can be a practical consideration in certain applications, and precautions are often taken to mitigate it.

DMSO's chemical structure, physical properties, and chemical properties are integral to its multifaceted nature and utility in research, industry, and medicine. Its remarkable solvency, reactivity, and stability make it a valuable and versatile compound with diverse applications across multiple fields. A thorough understanding of DMSO's science is essential for safe and effective utilization.

## 2.2 How DMSO Works

Understanding how DMSO (Dimethyl sulfoxide) works involves exploring its mechanisms of action, particularly in the context of its solvency and its ability to facilitate the transdermal absorption of various substances.

**Solvency and Dissolution:**

DMSO's primary function, and one of its most well-known attributes, is its exceptional solvency. It can dissolve a wide range of organic and inorganic substances, making it a valuable solvent in various fields, including chemistry and biology. This exceptional solvency is due to several key factors:

- **Polarity:** DMSO is a highly polar compound, with a sulfur-oxygen double bond and the ability to form hydrogen bonds.

This high polarity allows it to interact with a broad spectrum of compounds, including those that are both polar and nonpolar. As a result, DMSO can dissolve substances that might be insoluble in other common solvents like water.

- **Nucleophilicity:** DMSO can act as a nucleophile, meaning it can donate electrons to react with electrophilic species. This property allows DMSO to participate in various chemical reactions, making it a valuable reagent in organic synthesis.

- **Dissolving Ions:** DMSO can effectively dissolve ionic compounds, creating a medium for various chemical reactions and processes, such as ion transport and electrolysis.

- **Hydrophilic and Lipophilic:**
  DMSO is both hydrophilic
  (attracted to water) and
  lipophilic (attracted to lipids or
  fats). This dual nature
  contributes to its ability to
  dissolve a wide range of
  substances, including both
  hydrophilic and lipophilic
  molecules.

**Transdermal Absorption:**

DMSO's ability to facilitate the transdermal absorption of substances through the skin is another significant aspect of how it works, particularly in medical and pharmaceutical applications. This mechanism involves the following principles:

- **Enhanced Permeability:**
  DMSO is known for its
  capacity to increase the

permeability of biological membranes, including the skin. It can alter the properties of the skin, making it more permeable to certain compounds. This property has led to the exploration of DMSO as a transdermal carrier for drug delivery.

- **Selective Transport:** DMSO can transport specific substances through the skin. When combined with other compounds, it can enable the passage of drugs and therapeutic agents into the bloodstream, bypassing the gastrointestinal system and offering an alternative route for drug administration.

- **Applications:** DMSO's transdermal delivery

mechanism has been investigated in the treatment of various conditions, such as pain management and anti-inflammatory therapy. It has also been explored in the field of dermatology for the treatment of skin disorders.

It's important to note that while DMSO has demonstrated significant potential as a transdermal carrier, its use in this capacity is subject to regulatory considerations and safety concerns. The effectiveness and safety of DMSO in transdermal drug delivery depend on various factors, including the specific substance being delivered and the concentration of DMSO used.

DMSO works primarily as a solvent, with its exceptional solvency driven by its polarity, nucleophilicity, and unique properties. Additionally, its ability to enhance transdermal absorption has opened up new possibilities in medical and pharmaceutical applications. However, the use of DMSO in drug delivery must be carefully considered and regulated to ensure safety and efficacy.

## 2.3 Safety Considerations

Dimethyl sulfoxide (DMSO) is a versatile compound with numerous applications, but it also comes with specific safety considerations that must be understood and managed when handling and using it in various settings. Here are some key safety considerations associated with DMSO:

## 1. Skin and Eye Contact:

- **Skin Absorption:** DMSO is well-known for its ability to penetrate the skin. While this property can be useful for transdermal drug delivery, it also means that DMSO can carry contaminants or other substances into the body if it comes into contact with the skin. Always wear protective gloves and lab coats when handling DMSO, especially in concentrated form.

- **Eye Irritation:** DMSO can cause eye irritation and should be handled with care to prevent accidental contact with the eyes. Safety goggles should be worn when working with DMSO.

## 2. Inhalation:

- DMSO should be used in well-ventilated areas to avoid inhalation of its vapors. While DMSO is not considered highly toxic when inhaled, it can produce an unpleasant odor and cause respiratory irritation in high concentrations.

## 3. Storage and Handling:

- Store DMSO in appropriate containers, away from incompatible materials and in a cool, dry place. It should be kept in a tightly sealed container to prevent moisture absorption and contamination.

- Avoid storing DMSO near strong oxidizing agents, as it may react with them.

## 4. Material Compatibility:

- DMSO is an excellent solvent, but it may dissolve or react with some materials. Be cautious when selecting containers, equipment, and materials for use with DMSO, and ensure they are compatible to avoid accidents or contamination.

## 5. Chemical Stability:

- DMSO is generally stable, but it can degrade over time, especially when exposed to air. Check the integrity and purity of DMSO solutions before use, as degraded DMSO may contain impurities that could be harmful or affect experimental results.

## 6. Purity and Quality:

- When working with DMSO for research or medical purposes, ensure that you are using high-quality, pure DMSO. Impurities in low-quality DMSO can lead to unpredictable results or safety issues.

## 7. Regulations and Guidelines:

- Familiarize yourself with the regulations and guidelines related to the use of DMSO in your specific field or application. Different industries and research areas may have distinct requirements for handling and using DMSO.

## 8. Personal Protective Equipment (PPE):

- Always use appropriate personal protective equipment, including gloves, lab coats, safety goggles, and any other protective gear recommended in your workplace or laboratory safety protocols.

## 9. First Aid:

- In the event of skin contact, eye exposure, or accidental ingestion, follow the recommended first aid procedures. For severe cases or if any adverse symptoms occur, seek medical attention immediately.

## 10. Disposal:

- Dispose of DMSO and DMSO-contaminated materials in accordance with local regulations and guidelines. DMSO should not be poured down the drain unless it is specifically permitted by local

wastewater treatment
authorities.

Safety is of utmost importance when
working with DMSO, and it's crucial
to follow proper handling procedures
and safety protocols to minimize risks
and ensure the safe use of this
versatile solvent. Consulting safety
data sheets (SDS) and guidelines
provided by manufacturers and
regulatory agencies can provide
specific safety information for your
intended use of DMSO.

# CHAPTER 3

# Getting Started with DMSO

## 3.1 Handling and Storage

Handling and storing Dimethyl sulfoxide (DMSO) correctly is essential to ensure its integrity, safety, and effectiveness in various applications. DMSO is a versatile solvent with unique properties, and its characteristics require specific considerations when handling and storing.

**Handling DMSO:**

1. **Protective Gear:** Always wear appropriate personal protective equipment (PPE) when

handling DMSO. This should include lab coats, gloves, and safety goggles to prevent skin and eye contact.

2. **Skin Contact:** DMSO can penetrate the skin easily, so be cautious when handling it. Use nitrile or latex gloves, and change them regularly to avoid contamination. If you experience skin contact, wash the affected area with plenty of water.

3. **Eye Protection:** DMSO can cause eye irritation. Wear safety goggles or a face shield to shield your eyes when working with DMSO, and be prepared to rinse your eyes thoroughly with water if there is accidental contact.

4. **Ventilation:** Use DMSO in well-ventilated areas or under a fume hood. Adequate ventilation helps to reduce exposure to its vapors and unpleasant odor.

5. **Inhalation:** Avoid inhaling DMSO vapors. While DMSO is not highly toxic when inhaled, it can cause respiratory irritation. Keep containers tightly closed when not in use.

6. **Spills and Cleanup:** In the event of a spill, absorb DMSO with an inert material, such as dry sand or absorbent pads. Dispose of the contaminated material in accordance with local regulations.

**Storage of DMSO:**

1.  **Container Selection:** Store DMSO in appropriate containers made of materials that are compatible with it. Glass, high-density polyethylene (HDPE), or fluorinated containers are suitable choices. Ensure that the containers have a tight seal to prevent moisture absorption and contamination.

2.  **Cool, Dry Location:** Store DMSO in a cool, dry place away from direct sunlight and heat sources. Exposure to high temperatures can cause evaporation and degradation.

3.  **Moisture Control:** DMSO is hygroscopic, meaning it absorbs moisture from the air. Store it in a dry environment to

prevent dilution of the solution over time.

4. **Incompatible Materials:** Keep DMSO away from strong oxidizing agents, such as concentrated acids or chlorine compounds, as it may react with them.

5. **Labeling:** Clearly label containers with the contents, concentration, and date of preparation to avoid confusion and ensure safe handling.

6. **Segregation:** Store DMSO away from incompatible chemicals to prevent potential reactions or contamination.

7. **Regulations:** Be aware of and adhere to any local or workplace regulations

regarding the storage of chemicals, including DMSO.

8. **Quality Check:** Regularly inspect stored DMSO to ensure its purity and integrity. Over time, DMSO can degrade or absorb impurities, which can affect its performance.

By following these handling and storage guidelines, you can ensure the safe and effective use of DMSO in your laboratory, industry, or other applications. Proper handling and storage practices are crucial to maintaining the quality and safety of DMSO for its intended purposes.

# 3.2 Dilution and Concentration

Diluting and concentrating Dimethyl sulfoxide (DMSO) is a common practice in various applications, as it allows you to adjust the concentration of DMSO to suit your specific needs. Whether you need a more concentrated solution for a particular experiment or a less concentrated one for a specific application, understanding how to dilute and concentrate DMSO properly is essential.

**Diluting DMSO:**

1. **Safety Precautions:** Always wear appropriate personal protective equipment (PPE), such as lab coats, gloves, and safety goggles, when working

with DMSO, whether it's in its concentrated form or a dilution.

2. **Select a Solvent:** Choose a suitable solvent for diluting DMSO. Common solvents used for dilution include water, ethanol, or other organic solvents. Ensure that the chosen solvent is compatible with your intended application.

3. **Calculating the Desired Concentration:** Determine the concentration of the DMSO solution you wish to achieve. You can calculate the required volume of the concentrated DMSO and the solvent using the formula:

$$C_1V_1 = C_2V_2$$

- C1: Concentration of the concentrated DMSO solution.

- V1: Volume of the concentrated DMSO solution.

- C2: Desired concentration of the diluted DMSO solution.

- V2: Volume of the solvent to be added.

4. **Mixing:** Add the calculated volume of the concentrated DMSO solution to a container and then add the solvent while stirring continuously. Mixing ensures that the components are uniformly distributed, resulting in the desired concentration.

5. **Verification:** Use appropriate analytical techniques or tools to verify the concentration of the diluted DMSO solution if precision is critical for your application.

**Concentrating DMSO:**

1. **Safety Precautions:** Ensure you are following safety guidelines when handling concentrated DMSO.

2. **Select a Method:** Concentrating DMSO typically involves removing the solvent from a dilute solution to leave a more concentrated solution behind. Common methods for concentration include:

   - Evaporation: Place the DMSO solution in an open container and allow the solvent to evaporate. This method works well when working with non-volatile solvents.

- Distillation: Use distillation equipment to separate the solvent from the DMSO. This method is particularly useful when working with volatile solvents.

3. **Heat and Ventilation:** If using heat, apply it cautiously and ensure adequate ventilation to prevent inhaling DMSO vapors. Be aware that DMSO has a relatively high boiling point, so the process may take time.

4. **Monitoring Concentration:** Regularly check the concentration of DMSO during

the concentration process to prevent over-concentration, which may result in unwanted precipitation or crystallization.

5. **Safety and Regulations:** Adhere to safety protocols and local regulations when using methods that involve heat, open containers, or volatile solvents.

following these guidelines, you can effectively dilute and concentrate DMSO to achieve the desired concentration for your specific applications while maintaining safety and accuracy in your work.

# CHAPTER 4

# DMSO as a Solvent

## 4.1 Using DMSO as a Solvent

Dimethyl sulfoxide (DMSO) is renowned for its exceptional solvency and versatility as a solvent. It has the ability to dissolve a wide range of compounds, both polar and nonpolar, making it a valuable tool in various fields, including chemistry, biology, and industry. Here's how to effectively use DMSO as a solvent:

**1. Selection of DMSO:**

- Ensure you are working with high-quality, pure DMSO to maintain the integrity of your experiments or applications. Impure DMSO may contain contaminants that can affect your results.

## 2. Safety Precautions:

- Always prioritize safety. Wear appropriate personal protective equipment (PPE), including lab coats, gloves, and safety goggles, as DMSO can be absorbed through the skin and may cause eye irritation.

## 3. Compatibility Check:

- Before using DMSO as a solvent, ensure that your solute (the substance you want to dissolve) is compatible with DMSO. DMSO's unique properties make it a versatile solvent, but some substances may not dissolve or may react with it.

## 4. Determining the Concentration:

- Decide on the concentration of the DMSO solution you need for your application. This could range from highly concentrated to dilute, depending on the specific requirements of your experiment or process.

## 5. Measuring DMSO:

- Use precision measuring equipment to accurately dispense the required volume of DMSO. Ensure that your equipment is clean and free from any contaminants.

## 6. Dissolution Process:

- Place the solute into a container or beaker and add the

calculated volume of DMSO.
Stir or agitate the mixture to
facilitate dissolution.
Depending on the solute and
the concentration, this process
may take some time. If
necessary, provide gentle
heating, but be cautious to
avoid overheating and
evaporation.

## 7. Analysis and Verification:

- For precision work, consider
  analyzing the resulting solution
  using appropriate analytical
  techniques to confirm its
  concentration and purity. This
  is particularly crucial in
  research and analytical
  chemistry.

## 8. Temperature Considerations:

- Be mindful of the temperature at which you are working. DMSO has a relatively high boiling point (189°C or 372°F), so it is generally stable at higher temperatures. However, the temperature can affect the rate of dissolution and may be critical for certain solutes.

## 9. Compatibility with Materials:

- Consider the materials you use for containers, stirring rods, and other equipment. DMSO can dissolve or react with some materials, such as certain plastics. Glass or high-density polyethylene (HDPE) containers are often preferred.

## 10. Storage and Labeling:

- Store DMSO solutions in appropriate containers with

secure seals to prevent moisture absorption and contamination. Label containers with the contents, concentration, and date of preparation for future reference.

Using DMSO as a solvent offers a versatile and efficient way to dissolve a wide range of compounds for various applications. By following these guidelines, you can harness the solvency and flexibility of DMSO while ensuring the safety and precision of your work.

## 4.2 Mixing DMSO with Other Substances

Mixing Dimethyl sulfoxide (DMSO) with other substances is a common practice in various fields, including chemistry, biology, and medicine. DMSO's unique properties make it an effective solvent and carrier for a wide range of compounds. Here are the steps to effectively mix DMSO with other substances:

## 1. Safety Precautions:

- Always prioritize safety. Wear appropriate personal protective equipment (PPE), including lab coats, gloves, and safety goggles, when working with DMSO. Take precautions to prevent skin contact and eye irritation.

## 2. Compatibility Check:

- Ensure that the substances you intend to mix with DMSO are compatible. DMSO is a versatile solvent, but not all

compounds can be effectively
mixed or dissolved in it.

## 3. Proper Solvent Selection:

- Choose the appropriate solvent
  for your specific application.
  Depending on the solute, you
  may need to use water, ethanol,
  or other organic solvents in
  combination with DMSO. The
  choice of solvent can affect the
  solubility and stability of the
  mixture.

## 4. Determine the Concentration:

- Decide on the desired
  concentration of the final
  mixture. The concentration can
  vary depending on your
  specific needs and the solute's
  properties.

## 5. Measuring Substances:

- Accurately measure the quantities of DMSO and the other substances involved. Use precision equipment and ensure they are clean and free from contaminants.

## 6. Mixing Process:

- Place the solute (the substance you want to dissolve in DMSO) in a container or beaker. Add the calculated volume of DMSO and the other solvent if needed. Stir or agitate the mixture to facilitate dissolution.

## 7. Temperature Considerations:

- Be mindful of the temperature at which you are mixing. DMSO is stable at higher temperatures, but the temperature can affect the rate of dissolution and may be crucial for certain solutes.

## 8. Analysis and Verification:

- If precision and accuracy are paramount, consider using appropriate analytical techniques to confirm the concentration and purity of the final mixture. This is especially important in research and analytical chemistry.

## 9. Compatibility with Materials:

- Consider the materials used for containers, stirring rods, and other equipment. DMSO can dissolve or react with some materials, so choose glass or high-density polyethylene (HDPE) containers when appropriate.

## 10. Storage and Labeling:

- Store the mixture in appropriate containers with secure seals to prevent moisture absorption and contamination. Label containers with the contents, concentration, and date of preparation for future reference.

## 11. Documentation:

- Keep thorough records of the mixing process, including the precise amounts of substances used, the order of addition, and any specific conditions (e.g., temperature) during the process.

## 12. Testing and Verification:

- In some cases, it may be necessary to perform tests or assays to confirm that the mixture meets the desired specifications for your specific application.

following these guidelines, you can effectively mix DMSO with other substances to create solutions tailored to your research, industrial, or medical needs. Understanding the compatibility of the substances, selecting the appropriate solvents, and ensuring accurate measurements are essential for successful mixing with DMSO.

## 4.3 Compatibility with Different Compounds

Dimethyl sulfoxide (DMSO) is a versatile solvent known for its remarkable ability to dissolve a wide range of compounds. However, its compatibility with different substances can vary, and it's important to understand which compounds are suitable for mixing with DMSO and which may pose challenges. Here's a guide on the compatibility of DMSO with various types of compounds:

## 1. Organic Compounds:

- **Aliphatic Hydrocarbons:** Generally compatible with DMSO.

- **Aromatic Hydrocarbons:** Often soluble in DMSO, especially at elevated temperatures.

- **Alcohols:** Generally soluble in DMSO. The solubility increases with the polarity of the alcohol.

- **Aldehydes and Ketones:**
  Usually soluble in DMSO,
  especially at elevated
  temperatures.

- **Esters:** Often soluble in
  DMSO.

- **Carboxylic Acids:** Solubility
  may vary, with some
  carboxylic acids dissolving
  well in DMSO.

## 2. Inorganic Compounds:

- **Salts:** DMSO can dissolve
  various salts, including metal
  halides and other ionic
  compounds.

- **Acids:** DMSO can dissolve
  some acids, but compatibility
  varies depending on the
  specific acid and concentration.

- **Bases:** DMSO can dissolve bases to some extent, but this may depend on the base and concentration.

- **Metal Compounds:** Many metal salts are soluble in DMSO. However, compatibility can differ for different metals and ligands.

## 3. Biological Compounds:

- **Proteins and Enzymes:** DMSO can be used as a solvent for proteins and enzymes, although its compatibility depends on the protein and concentration. It can be particularly useful for protein storage and analysis.

- **Nucleic Acids (DNA, RNA):** DMSO is commonly used in molecular biology and is compatible with DNA and RNA. It can be used to facilitate the solubility and storage of these molecules.

## 4. Pharmaceuticals:

- **Many pharmaceutical compounds:** DMSO is used as a vehicle in drug formulations. It can enhance the solubility and bioavailability of certain drugs. However, compatibility varies among different drug compounds.

## 5. Polymers:

- **Some polymers:** DMSO can dissolve or swell some polymers. Compatibility depends on the specific polymer and its structure.

## 6. Incompatible Compounds:

- **Water-Insensitive Compounds:** DMSO can absorb moisture from the air, which may make it incompatible with water-sensitive compounds.

- **Highly Reactive Compounds:** DMSO's reactivity may not be suitable for highly reactive substances that could react with the solvent.

## 7. Solubility and Concentration:

- The solubility of compounds in DMSO can vary with concentration, temperature, and the specific characteristics of the solute. Solubility charts and guidelines are often available for reference.

## 8. Safety Considerations:

- Always handle DMSO and mixed solutions with appropriate safety precautions, especially if you're working with potentially hazardous or unknown compounds.

It's essential to conduct compatibility tests or refer to established literature and solubility data to determine the suitability of DMSO as a solvent for specific compounds. Additionally, consider the intended use of the mixture and whether the solute's properties align with your research or application goals.

# CHAPTER 5

# DMSO's Therapeutic Potential

Dimethyl sulfoxide (DMSO) has garnered significant attention for its therapeutic potential in various medical and pharmaceutical applications. Its unique properties, including its ability to penetrate biological membranes and solubilize a wide range of substances, have made it a versatile compound for different treatment modalities. Here are two key aspects of DMSO's therapeutic potential:

# 5.1 Medical and Pharmaceutical Applications

DMSO has found applications in the medical and pharmaceutical fields, demonstrating potential in various areas:

**a. Anti-Inflammatory and Analgesic Properties:**

- DMSO's anti-inflammatory properties have led to its investigation as a potential treatment for conditions like arthritis and muscle pain. It can be applied topically or through transdermal delivery methods to provide relief from inflammation and pain.

**b. Cryopreservation:**

- DMSO is widely used in the cryopreservation of cells, tissues, and stem cells. It helps protect biological materials during freezing and preserves their viability for future use in transplantation, research, and regenerative medicine.

### c. Drug Delivery:

- DMSO is employed as a solvent and carrier for various pharmaceutical compounds. It enhances the solubility of certain drugs, allowing for more effective and controlled drug delivery.

### d. Dermatological Conditions:

- DMSO has been studied for its potential in treating dermatological conditions, such as certain skin disorders and

scleroderma. Its ability to
penetrate the skin can make it a
vehicle for therapeutic agents.

## e. Bladder Disorders:

- In urology, DMSO has been
  used as a treatment for
  interstitial cystitis, a painful
  bladder condition. It is instilled
  directly into the bladder to
  alleviate symptoms.

## f. Vasodilation:

- DMSO can induce vasodilation,
  which may have applications in
  conditions characterized by
  reduced blood flow, such as
  Raynaud's disease.

# 5.2 Topical and Transdermal Uses

## a. Topical Pain Relief:

- DMSO is applied topically for localized pain relief, such as arthritis, muscle strains, or joint pain. It can provide rapid relief by reducing inflammation and increasing blood flow to the affected area.

## b. Transdermal Drug Delivery:

- DMSO's ability to enhance skin permeability makes it a valuable carrier for transdermal drug delivery. It can transport medications through the skin and into the bloodstream, allowing for systemic drug administration without the need for injections or oral ingestion.

## c. Skin Disorders:

- DMSO has been explored in the treatment of skin conditions, including burns, keloids, and scleroderma. Its use as a carrier for therapeutic agents can facilitate the treatment of these conditions.

## d. Cosmetic and Dermatological Products:

- DMSO is found in some cosmetic and dermatological products due to its skin-permeating properties. It can help improve the absorption of active ingredients in skincare products.

It's important to note that while DMSO offers therapeutic potential in these areas, its use in medical and pharmaceutical applications should be approached with caution and in accordance with established protocols and safety guidelines. Its effectiveness and safety can vary depending on the specific condition and formulation, and it may not be suitable for all patients or situations. Research and consultation with healthcare professionals are essential when considering the use of DMSO for therapeutic purposes.

## 5.3 Safety and Precautions in Therapeutic Applications

While Dimethyl sulfoxide (DMSO) has shown therapeutic potential in various applications, its use in medical and therapeutic contexts requires careful attention to safety and precautions due to its unique properties. Here are key safety considerations and precautions for therapeutic applications of DMSO:

## 1. Purity and Quality:

- Ensure that you are using high-quality, pure DMSO in therapeutic applications. Impurities in DMSO can affect its effectiveness and safety.

## 2. Dosage and Concentration:

- Determine the appropriate dosage and concentration for the specific condition being treated. Consult with a healthcare professional to establish safe and effective dosing guidelines.

### 3. Skin Sensitivity:

- Be aware that DMSO can cause skin irritation in some individuals. Perform a patch test on a small area of skin to check for any adverse reactions before applying DMSO more broadly.

### 4. Safety Gear:

- When handling DMSO for therapeutic use, always wear appropriate personal protective equipment (PPE), including gloves and safety goggles.

### 5. Dilution and Formulation:

- Dilute DMSO as necessary to achieve the desired concentration for therapeutic applications. Ensure that you

are using a compatible solvent
for dilution.

## 6. Application Area:

- Apply DMSO topically only to
the intended area of treatment.
Avoid contact with eyes,
mucous membranes, or
sensitive skin areas.

## 7. Precautions for Sensitive Populations:

- Exercise caution when using
DMSO on children, pregnant or
nursing individuals, and people
with pre-existing medical
conditions. Consult a healthcare
professional for guidance in
such cases.

## 8. Allergic Reactions:

- Be vigilant for signs of allergic
reactions, such as rash, itching,

or swelling, which may indicate sensitivity to DMSO. Discontinue use if allergic reactions occur.

## 9. Monitoring and Assessment:

- Regularly assess the progress and impact of DMSO treatment on the condition being treated. Adjust the treatment plan as necessary based on the individual's response.

## 10. Adverse Effects:

- Be aware of potential side effects and adverse reactions associated with DMSO, such as skin dryness or a garlic-like odor. If any adverse effects are observed, consult a healthcare professional.

## 11. Avoiding Contamination:

- Prevent the contamination of DMSO solutions with microorganisms, chemicals, or other impurities. Use sterilized containers and equipment.

## 12. Storage:

- Store DMSO solutions in tightly sealed, labeled containers in a cool, dry place, away from direct sunlight. Ensure that the containers are properly marked to prevent mix-ups.

## 13. Regulatory Compliance:

- Ensure compliance with local and national regulations governing the use of DMSO in therapeutic applications, especially in clinical settings.

## 14. Professional Guidance:

- In clinical or medical applications, consult with healthcare professionals who have experience with DMSO to ensure proper use and safety.

## 15. Research and Documentation:

- Maintain detailed records of treatment protocols, dosages, patient responses, and any adverse events for reference and future use.

## 16. Patient Informed Consent:

- Obtain informed consent from patients or participants when using DMSO in therapeutic applications, ensuring that they understand the potential risks and benefits.

Therapeutic use of DMSO should be approached with care, and the guidance of healthcare professionals is essential. DMSO may have the potential to provide relief in various conditions, but safety should always be a top priority when considering its application in a therapeutic context.

# CHAPTER 6

# DMSO in Research and Industry

Dimethyl sulfoxide (DMSO) plays a significant role in both scientific research and various industrial applications due to its exceptional solvency and versatile properties.

## 6.1 Scientific Research and Lab Applications

DMSO is a valuable tool in scientific research, providing solutions for a wide range of laboratory applications:

**a. Solvent in Chemistry and Biochemistry:**

- DMSO is a versatile solvent used in various chemical and biochemical processes. Its high solvency allows it to dissolve both polar and nonpolar compounds, making it essential for dissolving and preparing solutions of various reagents and compounds.

**b. Cryopreservation:**

- DMSO is widely used in the preservation of biological samples, cells, tissues, and stem cells. It serves as a cryoprotectant, preventing damage during freezing and ensuring the viability of biological materials for future use in research, medicine, and biotechnology.

**c. Cell Culture:**

- In cell biology, DMSO is used to cryopreserve and store cell lines. It can also facilitate the uptake of certain substances into cells, making it a valuable tool for molecular and cellular studies.

## d. Drug Delivery and Formulation:

- DMSO is employed in drug research and pharmaceutical development to enhance the solubility of poorly water-soluble drugs. It serves as a vehicle for drug delivery, aiding in the development of new drug formulations and improving bioavailability.

## e. DNA and RNA Research:

- DMSO is commonly used in molecular biology and genetics to prepare DNA and RNA samples, promote denaturation or hybridization, and facilitate the dissolution of nucleic acids.

## f. Analytical Chemistry:

- DMSO is used as a solvent and diluent in analytical chemistry techniques such as nuclear magnetic resonance (NMR) spectroscopy and high-performance liquid chromatography (HPLC) for the analysis of various compounds.

## g. Chemical Synthesis:

- DMSO's unique properties, including its nucleophilic nature, make it a valuable reagent for chemical synthesis and organic reactions.

# 6.2 Industrial and Manufacturing Uses

DMSO finds various applications in industrial and manufacturing processes:

## a. Paints and Coatings:

- DMSO is used in the formulation of paints, coatings, and inks due to its solvency and ability to dissolve and disperse various pigments and resins.

## b. Adhesives and Sealants:

- In the adhesive industry, DMSO is used as a solvent for various adhesive formulations, improving their bonding properties.

## c. Electronics and Semiconductor Manufacturing:

- DMSO is employed as a solvent and cleaning agent in semiconductor manufacturing and electronics industry for photoresist stripping and other applications.

## d. Polymer and Plastic Production:

- DMSO is used in the production of polymers, plastics, and resins due to its solvency and compatibility with a range of polymer materials.

## e. Metal Processing:

- In the metalworking industry, DMSO is used for cleaning and degreasing metal surfaces and as a component in metalworking fluids.

## f. Pharmaceuticals and Cosmetics:

- DMSO may be used in certain pharmaceutical formulations and cosmetic products, primarily as a solubilizing agent for active ingredients.

## g. Solvent Extraction:

- DMSO is utilized in solvent extraction processes, such as the purification of certain chemicals or the extraction of valuable compounds from raw materials.

## h. Textile and Leather Processing:

- DMSO can be used in textile dyeing and leather processing, aiding in the solubilization and application of dyes and chemicals.

DMSO's unique solvency and versatility make it a valuable resource in various scientific research, laboratory applications, and industrial processes. Its applications span a wide range of fields, from molecular biology to manufacturing, due to its ability to dissolve and transport a diverse array of substances.

## 6.3 Environmental Considerations

Dimethyl sulfoxide (DMSO) is a versatile solvent with numerous applications in research and industry. While it offers various benefits, its environmental impact and considerations must also be taken into account. Here are some key environmental factors to consider when using DMSO in different applications:

## 1. Biodegradability:

- DMSO is not readily biodegradable in the environment, which means it can persist in water and soil. This persistence may lead to long-term environmental concerns. Special care should be taken to prevent the release of DMSO into natural ecosystems.

## 2. Ecotoxicity:

- Studies have shown that DMSO may have adverse effects on aquatic organisms when discharged into water bodies. It can impact aquatic life and ecosystems, which underscores the importance of responsible handling and disposal.

## 3. Waste Disposal:

- Proper disposal of DMSO and DMSO-containing waste is critical. It should not be discharged into sewers or surface waters unless it is in compliance with local regulations and wastewater treatment guidelines. Waste containing DMSO should be managed and disposed of according to applicable environmental regulations.

## 4. VOC Emissions:

- DMSO can contribute to volatile organic compound (VOC) emissions, which can have air quality and environmental implications. Employing containment and capture systems, as well as implementing proper ventilation, can help reduce emissions in industrial settings.

## 5. Environmental Regulations:

- Compliance with local, regional, and national environmental regulations is essential when using DMSO in industrial processes or research. These regulations may specify permissible emission levels, waste disposal methods, and other environmental standards.

## 6. Alternatives and Reduction:

- Consider the use of alternative solvents or greener technologies when feasible. Reducing the overall use of DMSO or opting for environmentally friendly substitutes can help minimize its environmental impact.

## 7. Recycling and Recovery:

- In some cases, DMSO can be recovered and recycled, reducing the amount of solvent that needs to be disposed of as waste. Investigate the feasibility of recovery processes for your specific applications.

## 8. Safety Data Sheets (SDS):

- Refer to the safety data sheet (SDS) provided by the manufacturer for detailed information on the environmental hazards and safe disposal procedures for the specific DMSO product you are using.

## 9. Research Protocols:

- In research settings, evaluate whether the use of DMSO can be optimized to minimize environmental impact. This may involve using smaller quantities or finding ways to reduce solvent use in experiments.

## 10. Education and Training:

- Ensure that individuals handling DMSO in research or industrial settings are adequately trained in safety and environmental practices. Educating personnel on proper disposal and environmental considerations is essential.

Balancing the benefits of DMSO with its potential environmental impact is essential for responsible use. Adhering to established environmental regulations, reducing waste and emissions, and exploring more sustainable practices are key strategies to minimize the ecological footprint associated with DMSO usage in research and industry.

www.ingramcontent.com/pod-product-compliance
Lightning Source LLC
Chambersburg PA
CBHW050837260726
48660CB00006B/2287